Thank You!

AUTHOR'S NOTE

THANK YOU FOR CHOOSING THIS RECIPE BOOK!
I HOPE THAT YOU ENJOY MAKING AND EATING ALL OF THESE DELICIOUS CHEESECAKES. I KNOW I DID :)

I WANTED TO CREATE A YUMMY CHEESECAKE THAT WAS LIGHTER AND THAT PROVIDED MORE NUTRIENTS THAN A TRADITIONAL CHEESECAKE. SO THIS IS WHAT I CAME UP WITH! ALL THE RECIPES ARE ALSO GLUTEN- FREE!

COOKING A CHEESECAKE IN A PRESSURE COOKER IS A GREAT DECISION! IT ALLOWS THE CHEESECAKE TO COOK PERFECTLY AND AVOIDS USING A WATER BATH IN THE OVEN. BE SURE TO REVIEW THE TIPS & TRICKS SECTION BELOW.

TIPS & TRICKS

- SPRAY THE CHEESECAKE PAN WITH NONSTICK COOKING SPRAY BEFORE ADDING THE CRUST.
- WRAP THE OUTSIDE OF THE PAN IN ALUMINUM FOIL. THIS HELPS PREVENT WATER FROM LEAKING IN.
- COVER THE TOP OF THE CHEESECAKE WITH ALUMINUM FOIL. THIS PREVENTS WATER FROM DRIPPING ONTO THE CHEESECAKE.
- FILL THE BOTTOM OF THE PRESSURE COOKER WITH 1 C WATER. THE PRESSURE COOKER NEEDS WATER TO BUILD UP PRESSURE.
- USE A TRIVET, ALUMINUM FOIL BALLS, OR OTHER DEVICE TO ELEVATE THE CHEESECAKE SO IT IS NOT SITTING IN THE WATER.
- LET THE PRESSURE RELEASE NATURALLY. THIS IS COMPLETE WHEN THE SILVER PIN DROPS DOWN ON ITS OWN.
- USE A PAPER TOWEL TO DAB AWAY ANY EXTRA MOISTURE FROM ON TOP OF THE CHEESECAKE AFTER IT HAS FINISHED COOKING.
- LET THE CHEESECAKE COOL COMPLETELY AND REFRIGERATE IT BEFORE EATING. 8 HOURS MINIMUM BUT OVERNIGHT IS BEST!
- IF YOUR SEAL IS LOOSER, YOU MAY NEED TO ADD 5 MINUTES TO THE COOK TIME. IF THE CHEESECAKE IS SUPER LIQUIDY AFTER 35 MINUTES AND A NATURAL RELEASE, JUST PRESSURE COOK FOR 5 MORE MINUTES PLUS ANOTHER NATURAL RELEASE.

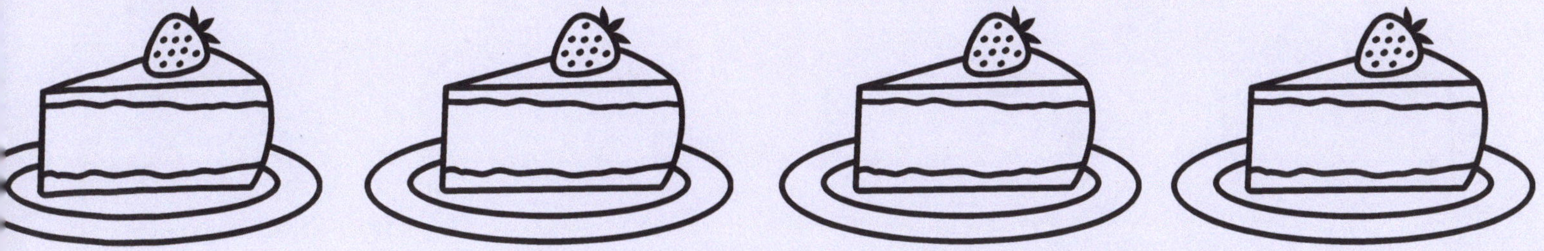

Table of Contents

- The Original Cheesecake
- Simple Fruit Jam
- Cookie Dough
- Cookie Dough Cheesecake
- Peanut Butter Cheesecake
- Cinnamon Cheesecake with Pumpkin Spice Swirl
- Carrot Cake Cheesecake
- cream cheese frosting
- Turtle Cheesecake
- Nut Caramel
- Chocolate Dream Cheesecake
- Chocolate cream cheese frosting
- Lemon Poppy Seed Cheesecake
- Chocolate Peppermint Cheesecake
- Gingerbread Cheesecake

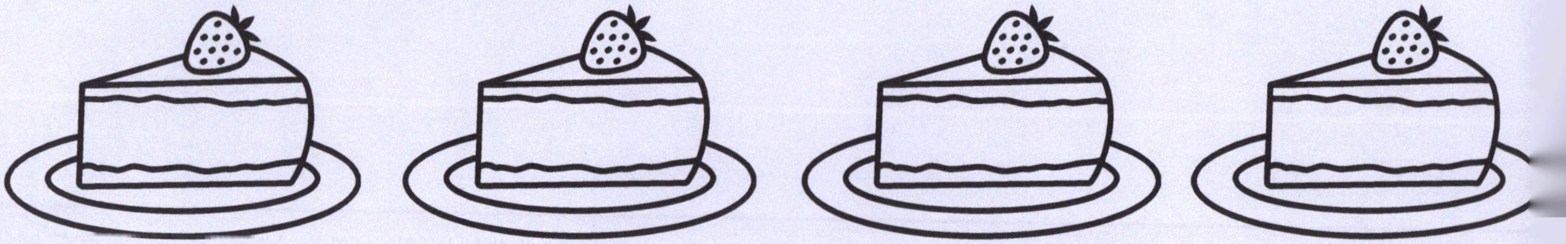

The OG

Original creamy cheesecake topped with all natural fruit jam. This is the best way to begin a cheesecake journey.

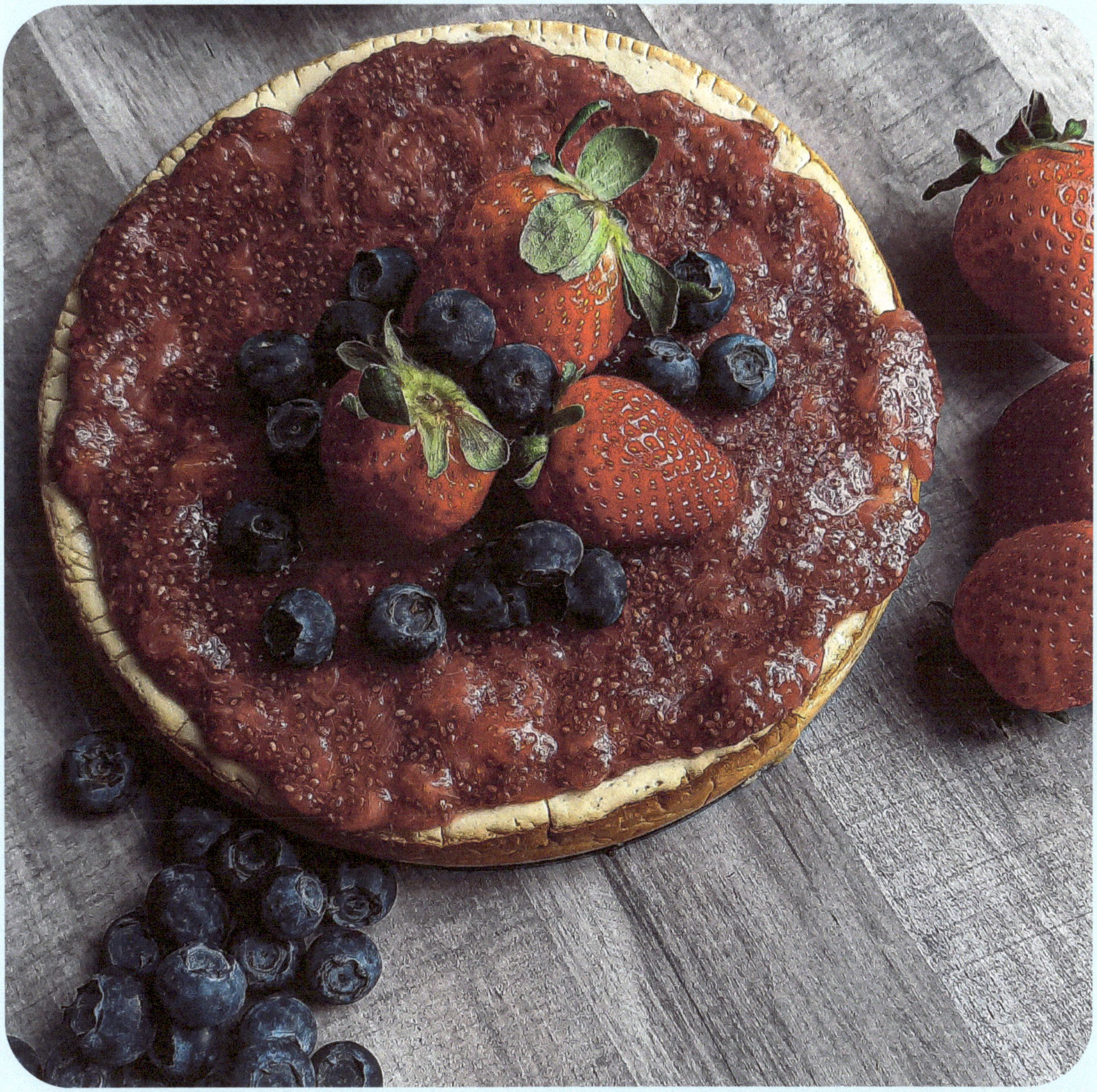

The OG

Crust Ingredients:

- 2/3 c quick oats
- 1 tbsp honey
- 2 tbsp water

Crust Method:

- Stir all ingredients together
- Spray pan with oil
- Press crust into pan
- Wrap the bottom of the pan in a double layer of aluminum foil

Cheesecake Ingredients:

- 1c cottage cheese
- 8 oz fat free cream cheese
- 1/2 c vanilla greek yogurt
- 2 eggs
- 1/4 c honey
- 1 tbsp oats
- 1 tsp vanilla extract

Cheesecake Method:

- Add all ingredients to a food processor and blend until smooth
- Pour cheesecake batter onto crust
- Cover cheesecake with aluminum foil
- Add water, lifting rack, and then cheesecake to pressure cooker
- Pressure cook on high for 35 minutes
- Wait for the pressure pin to release naturally
- Let cheesecake cool and refrigerate 8 hours or overnight before serving

simple fruit jam

INGREDIENTS:

- 2 c berries of choice, fresh or frozen
- 1 tbsp honey
- 3 tbsp chia seeds

METHOD:

- Place berries and honey in a saucepan and heat up on the stovetop
- Mash the berries
- Once they begin to boil, remove from heat
- Stir in chia seeds
- Let sit until the jam has thickened
- Refrigerate

ASSEMBLY:

- Top cheesecake with jam
- Devour :)

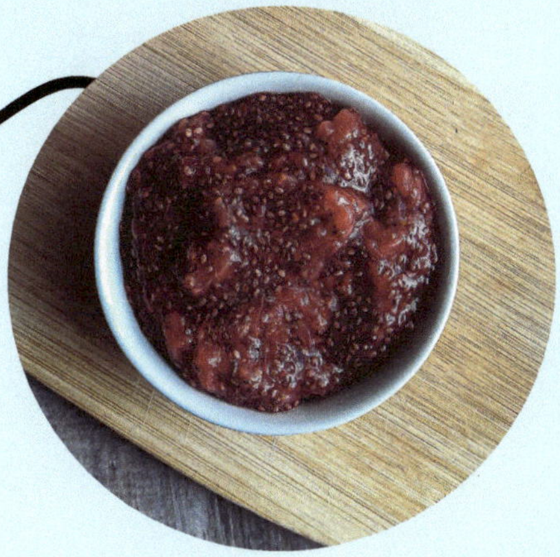

COOKIE DOUGH CHEESECAKE

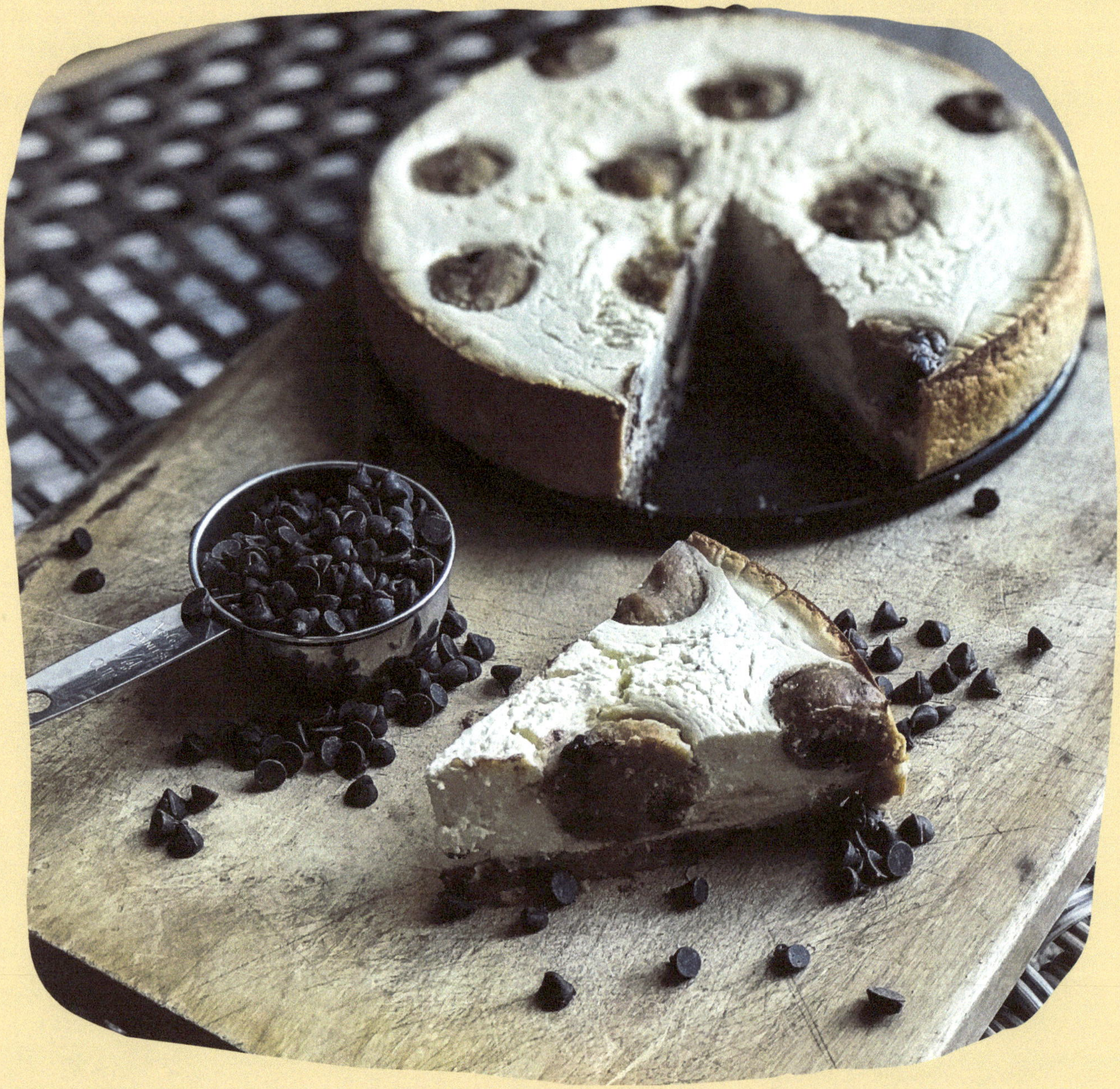

Two desserts in one?

Sign me up!

COOKIE DOUGH

Cookie Dough Recipe* :

- 1can drained and rinsed chickpeas
- 1/4 c milk of choice
- 1/2 c honey
- 2 tbsp nut butter (I used peanut butter)
- 1/2 c oats
- 1 tsp vanilla extract
- 1/4 c coconut flour
- chocolate chips or other mix-ins of choice (measure with your heart)

Cookie Dough Method:

- Add all ingredients except coconut flour and mix-ins to a food processor, blend until combined
- Fold in coconut flour and mix-ins
- Devour :)

Crust Method:

- Spray pan with oil
- Press about half of the cookie dough onto the bottom of the pan
- Save the rest to make balls to mix into the cheesecake
- Wrap the outside of the pan in a double layer of aluminum foil

*This cookie dough is a no-bake treat that can be enjoyed on its own too!

COOKIE DOUGH CHEESECAKE

Ingredients:

- 1 c cottage cheese
- 8 oz fat free cream cheese
- 1/2 c vanilla greek yogurt
- 2 eggs
- 1/4 c honey
- 1 tbsp oats
- 1 tsp vanilla extract

Method:

- Add all ingredients to a food processor and blend until smooth
- Pour cheesecake batter onto crust
- Drop balls of cookie dough into batter
- Cover cheesecake with aluminum foil
- Add water, lifting rack, and then cheesecake to pressure cooker
- Pressure cook on high for 35 minutes
- Wait for the pressure pin to release naturally
- Let cheesecake cool and refrigerate 8 hours or overnight before serving

Assembly:

- Top with melted chocolate if desired
- Devour :)

Peanut Butter Cheesecake

Calling all peanut butter lovers! This cheesecake is for you!

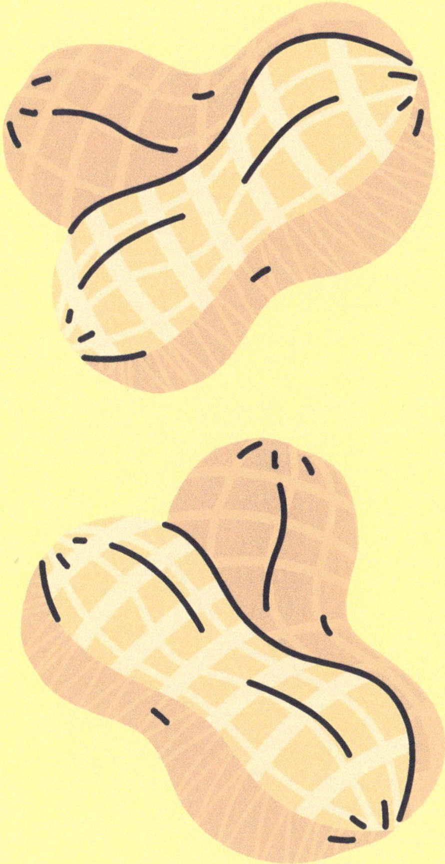

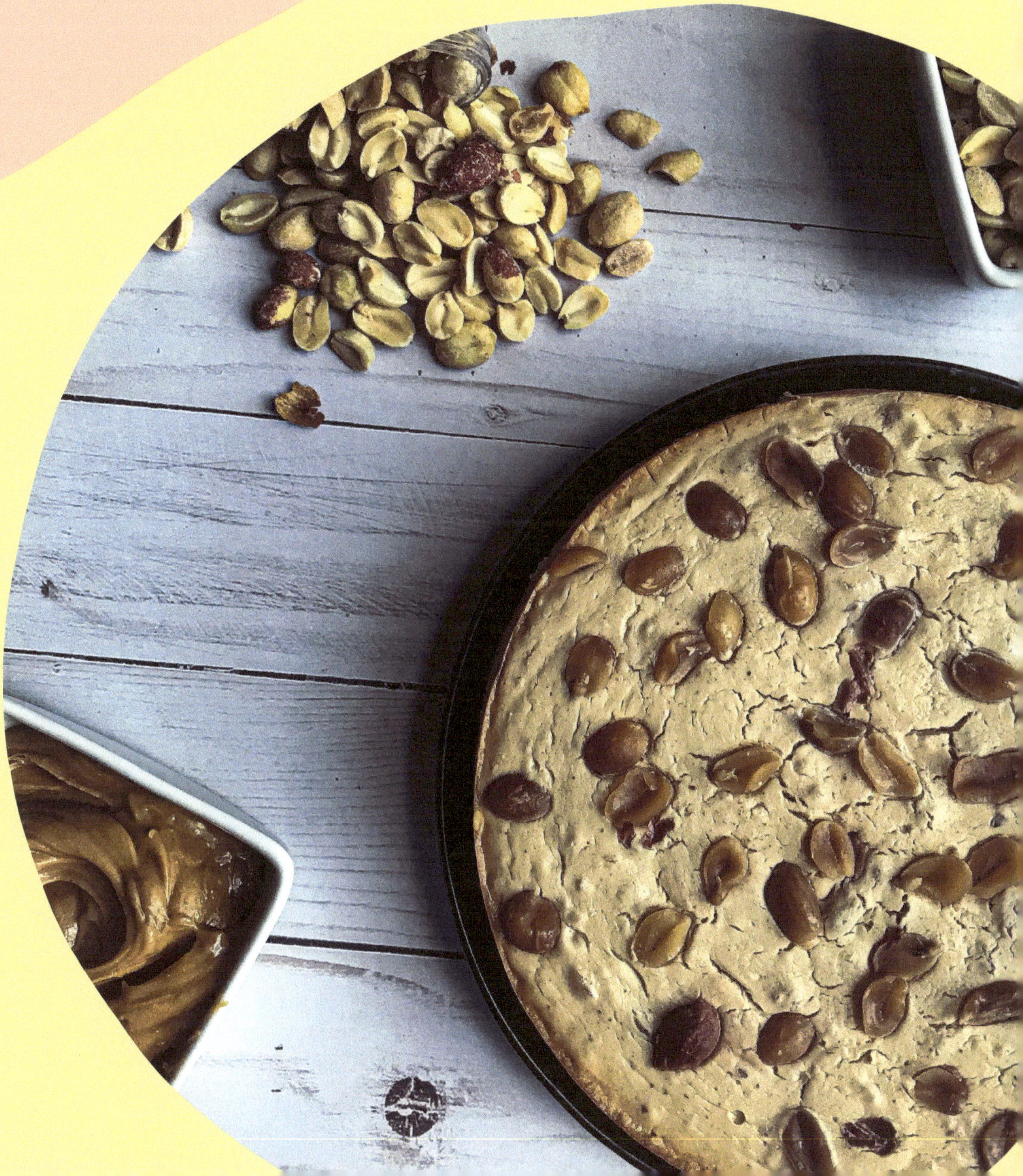

Peanut Butter Cheesecake

Crust Ingredients:

- 1/2 c quick oats
- 1/4 c dry roasted peanuts
- 1 tbsp honey
- 3 tbsp water

Crust Method:

- Pulse peanuts in food processor until crushed
- Stir all ingredients together
- Spray pan with oil
- Press crust into pan
- Wrap the bottom of the pan in a double layer of aluminum foil

Cheesecake Ingredients:

- 1 c cottage cheese
- 8 oz fat free cream cheese
- 1/2 c vanilla greek yogurt
- 2 eggs
- 1/4 c honey
- 1 tbsp oats
- 1 tsp vanilla extract
- 1/4 c creamy peanut butter
- 1/2 c dry roasted peanuts*

*You can omit the peanuts if you prefer no chunks in the cheesecake

Cheesecake Method:

- Add all ingredients except peanuts to a food processor and blend until smooth
- Add in peanuts and pulse until crushed
- Pour cheesecake batter onto crust
- Sprinkle additional peanuts on top
- Cover cheesecake with aluminum foil
- Add water, lifting rack, and then cheesecake to pressure cooker
- Pressure cook on high for 35 minutes
- Wait for the pressure pin to release naturally
- Let cheesecake cool and refrigerate 8 hours or overnight before serving
- Devour :)

Cinnamon Cheesecake w/ Pumpkin Spice Swirl

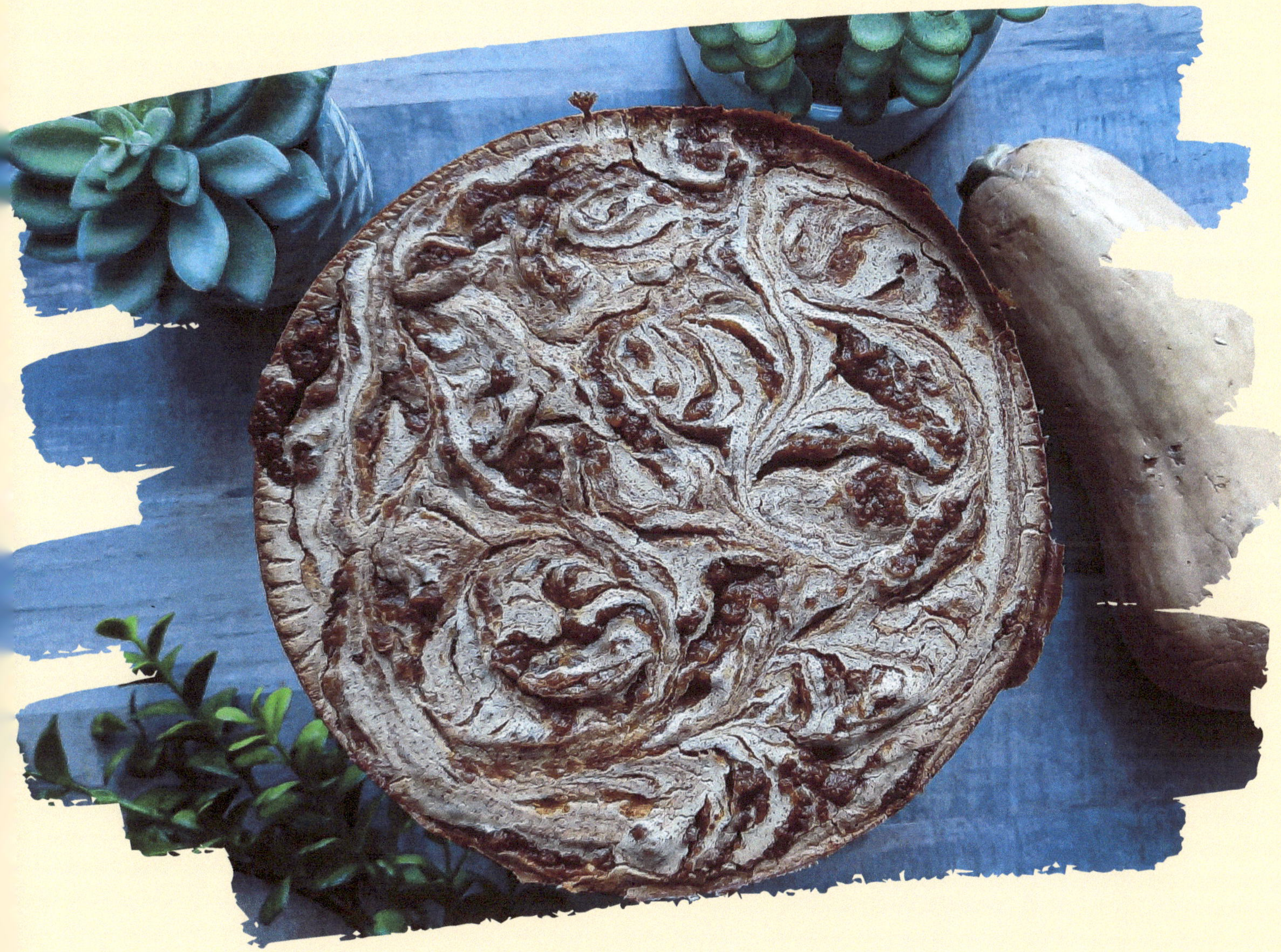

PERFECT FOR FALL -
OR REALLY ANY TIME OF YEAR :)

Cinnamon Cheesecake w/ Pumpkin Spice Swirl

CRUST RECIPE:

- 2/3 c quick oats
- 1 tsp cinnamon
- 1 tbsp honey
- 2 tbsp water

CRUST METHOD:

- Stir all ingredients together
- Spray pan with oil
- Press crust into pan
- Wrap the bottom of the pan in a double layer of aluminum foil

PUMPKIN SPICE SWIRL RECIPE:

- 2/3 c pumpkin puree
- 1 tsp pumpkin pie spice
- 2 tbsp honey

CHEESECAKE RECIPE:

- 1 c cottage cheese
- 8 oz fat free cream cheese
- 1/2 c vanilla greek yogurt
- 2 eggs
- 1/4 c honey
- 1 tbsp oats
- 1 tsp vanilla extract
- 1 tbsp cinnamon

CHEESECAKE METHOD:

- Add all cheesecake ingredients to a food processor and blend until smooth
- In a separate bowl, mix pumpkin spice swirl ingredients together
- Pour cheesecake batter onto crust
- Plop scoops of the pumpkin spice swirl onto the cheesecake and swirl with a knife
- Cover cheesecake with aluminum foil
- Add water, lifting rack, and then cheesecake to pressure cooker
- Pressure cook on high for 35 minutes
- Wait for the pressure pin to release naturally
- Let cheesecake cool and refrigerate 8 hours or overnight before serving

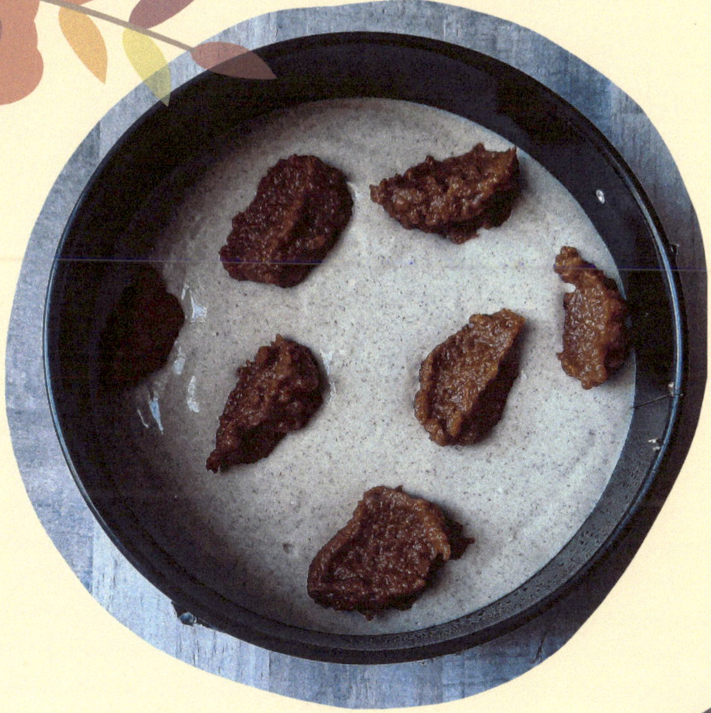

Add spoons of pumpkin

Swirl with a knife

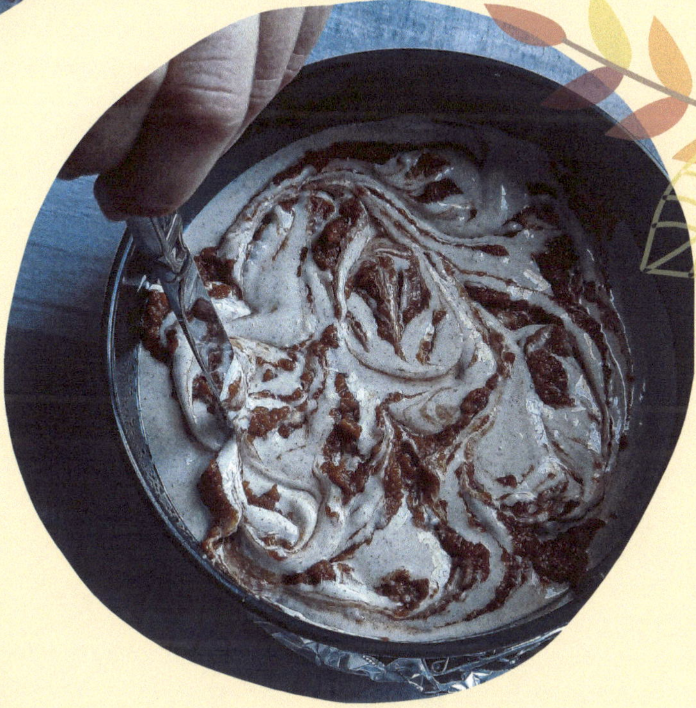

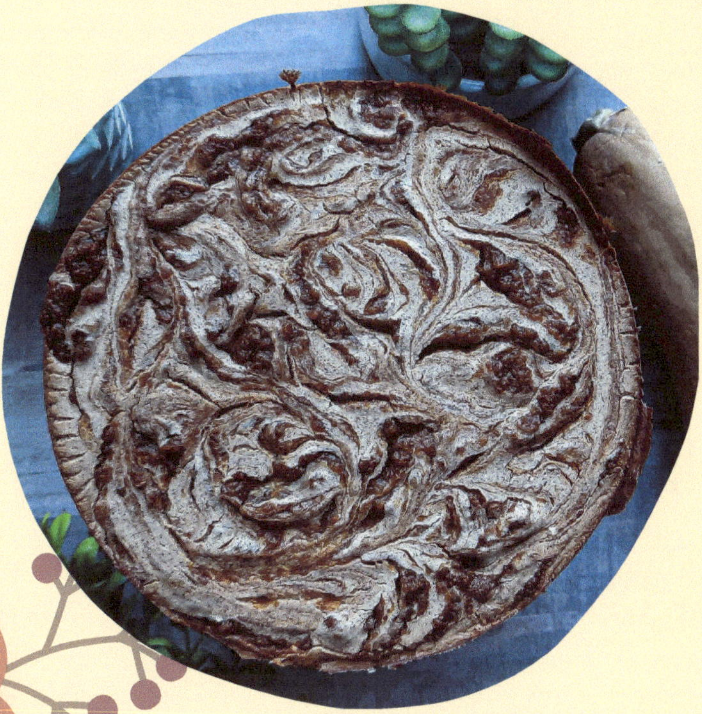

Cook, then Devour :)

Carrot Cake Cheesecake

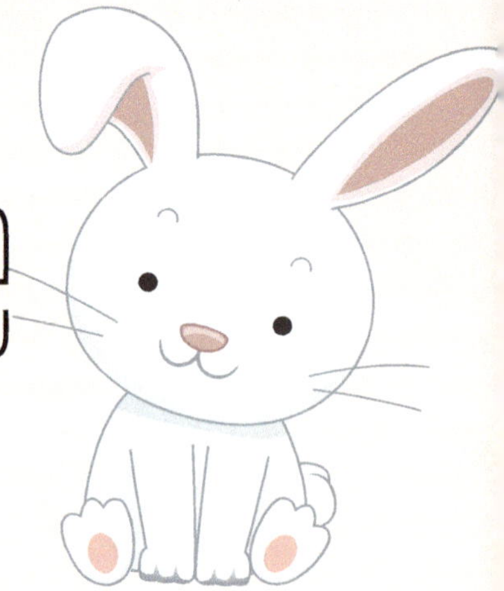

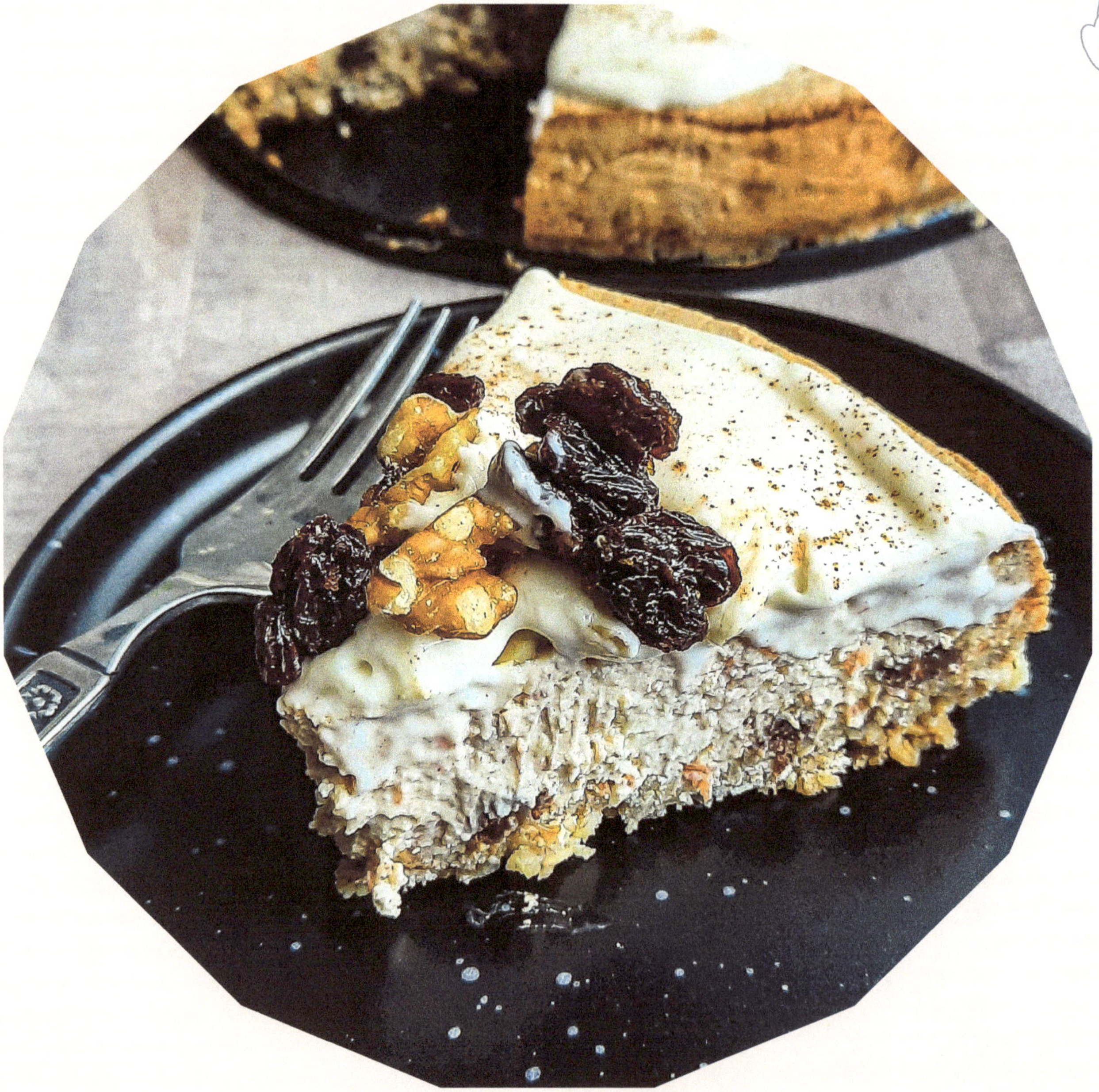

This classic cake flavor is even more delicious in cheesecake form!

Carrot Cake Cheesecake

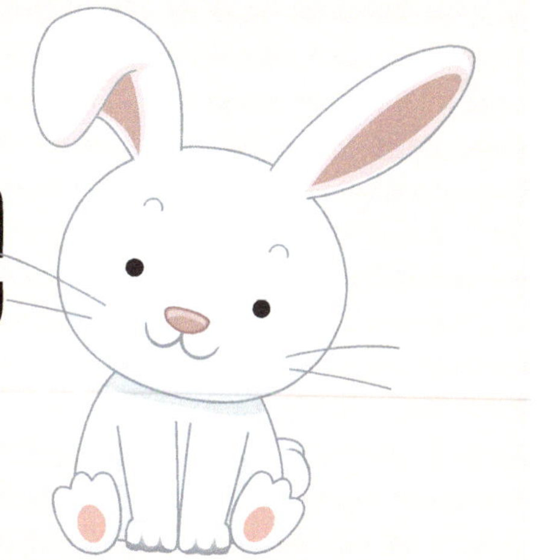

Crust Recipe:

- 2/3 c quick oats
-1 tsp cinnamon
- 1 tbsp honey
- 2 tbsp water

Crust Method:

- Stir all ingredients together
- Spray pan with oil
- Press crust into pan
- Wrap the bottom of the pan in a double layer of aluminum foil

Cheesecake Recipe:

- 1 c cottage cheese
- 8 oz fat free cream cheese
- 1/2 c vanilla greek yogurt
- 2 eggs
- 1/4 c honey
- 1 tbsp oats
- 1 tsp vanilla extract
- 1/3 c shredded carrot
-1/4 c raisins
- 1/4 c chopped walnuts
- 1 tsp cinnamon
- 1/4 tsp ginger
- 1/4 tsp nutmeg

Cheesecake Method:

- Add all ingredients except carrot, raisins, and walnuts to a food processor and blend until smooth
- Stir in carrot, raisins, and walnuts
- Pour cheesecake batter onto crust
- Cover cheesecake with aluminum foil
- Add water, lifting rack, and then cheesecake to pressure cooker
- Pressure cook on high for 35 minutes
- Wait for the pressure pin to release naturally
- Let cheesecake cool and refrigerate 8 hours or overnight before serving

Cream Cheese Frosting

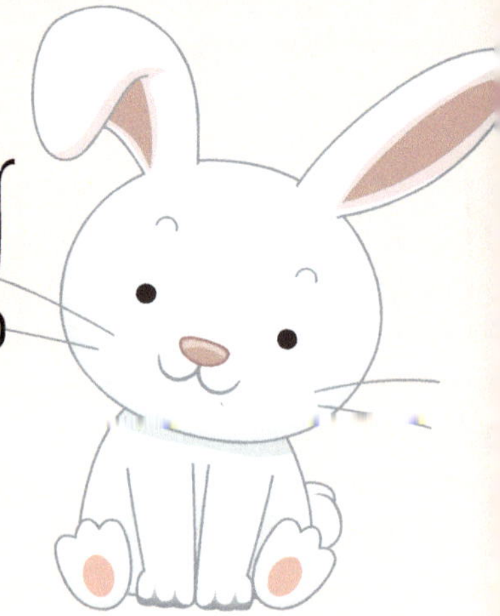

Cream Cheese Frosting Recipe:

- 8 oz fat free cream cheese
-1 c to1 1/2 c confectioners sugar (can adjust to your desired sweetness level)

Frosting Method:

- Use a hand mixer to beat cream cheese
- While beating, add in sugar a little at a time
- Refrigerate

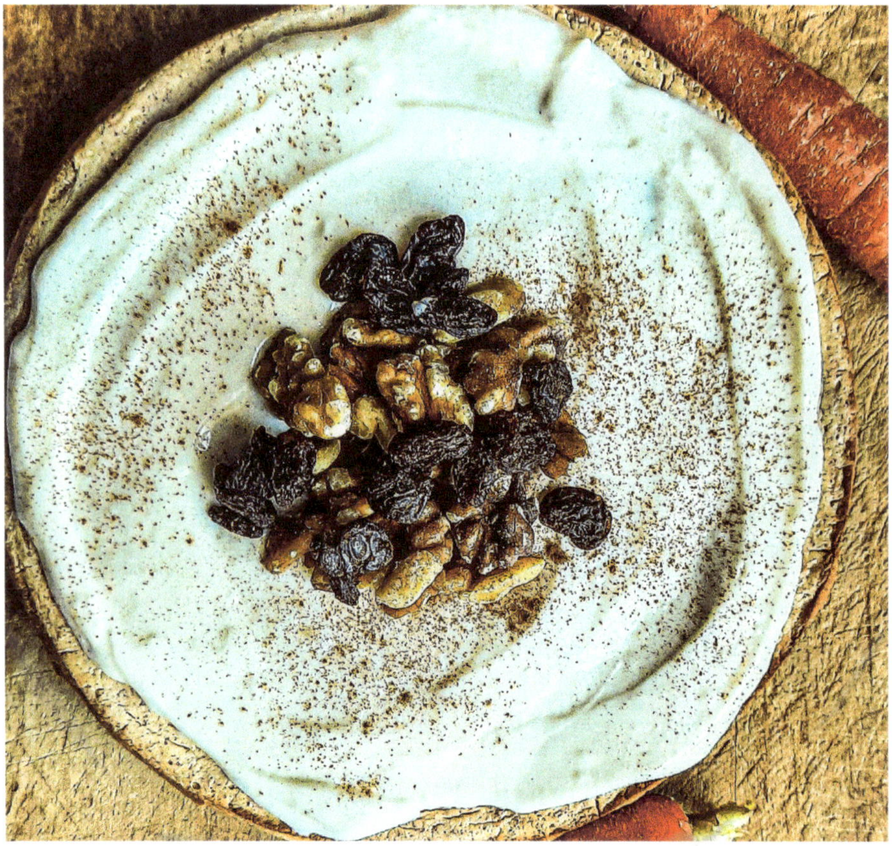

Assembly:

- Ice cheesecake with frostin
- Top with extra dried fruit, nuts, and cinnamon
-Devour :)

Turtle Cheesecake

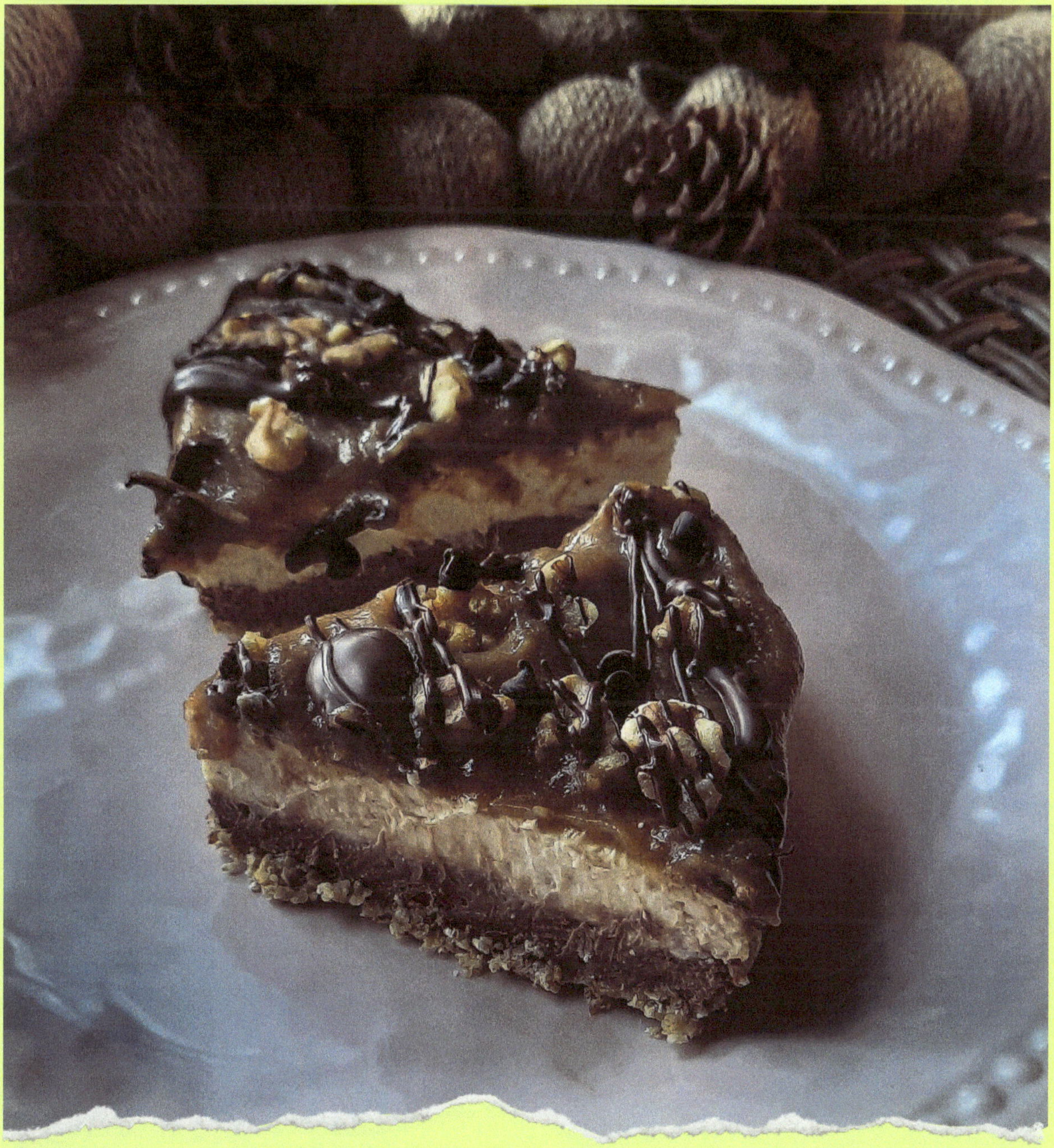

CHOCOLATE, CARAMEL, NUTS.

NEED I SAY MORE?

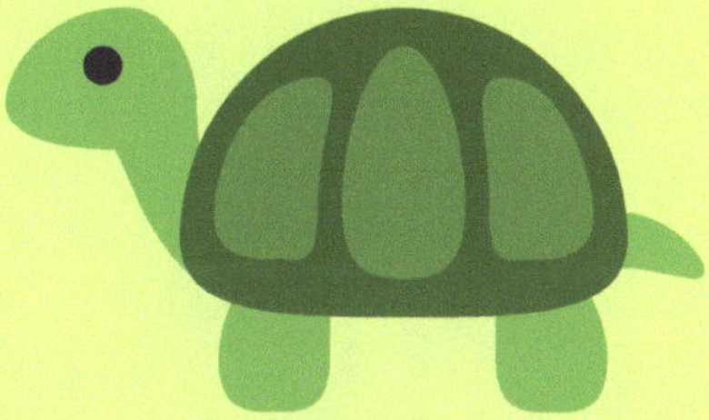

Turtle Cheesecake

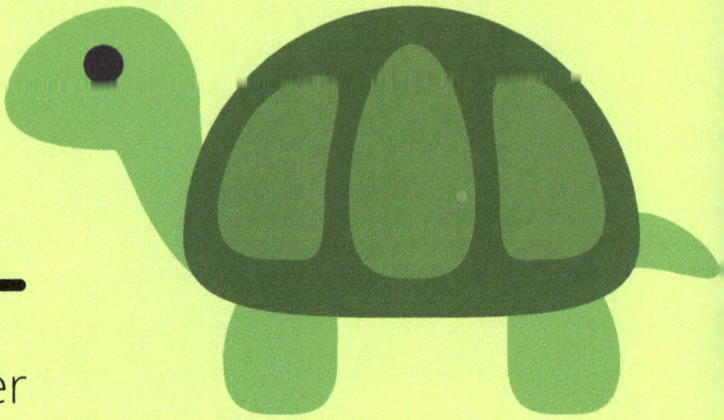

CRUST RECIPE:

- 2/3 c quick oats
- 1 tbsp honey
- 2 tbsp water

CRUST METHOD:

- Stir all ingredients together
- Spray pan with oil
- Press crust into pan
- Wrap the bottom of the pan in a double layer of aluminum foil

CHEESECAKE RECIPE:

- 1 c cottage cheese
- 8 oz fat free cream cheese
- 1/2 c vanilla greek yogurt
- 2 eggs
- 1/4 c honey
- 1 tbsp oats
- 1 tsp vanilla extract
- 1/4 c chocolate chips, melted (I used dark chocolate)

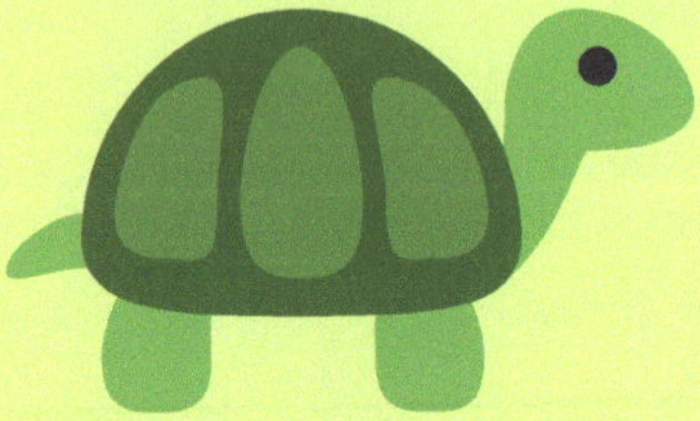

CHEESECAKE METHOD:

- Add all ingredients except melted chocolate to a food processor and blend
- Divide the batter in half
- Add the melted chocolate to one half of the batter and blend again to combine
- Pour the chocolate cheesecake batter onto crust
- Pour the regular cheesecake batter on top of the chocolate cheesecake batter
- Cover cheesecake with aluminum foil
- Add water, lifting rack, and then cheesecake to pressure cooker
- Pressure cook on high for 35 minutes
- Wait for the pressure pin to release naturally
- Let cheesecake cool and refrigerate 8 hours or overnight before serving

Nut Caramel

CARAMEL RECIPE:

-1 c dates
Warm water to soak dates in
- 1/2 c milk
- 1 tbsp honey
- 1/3 c chopped nut of choice (I used walnuts)

CARAMEL METHOD:

-Soak the dates in warm water for 10 mins
-Remove dates from water
-Add the dates, milk, and honey to a food processor and blend
-Stir the chopped nuts into the caramel
-Refrigerate

ASSEMBLY:

- Add the nut caramel mixture on top of the cheesecake
- Drizzle with melted chocolate
- Devour :)

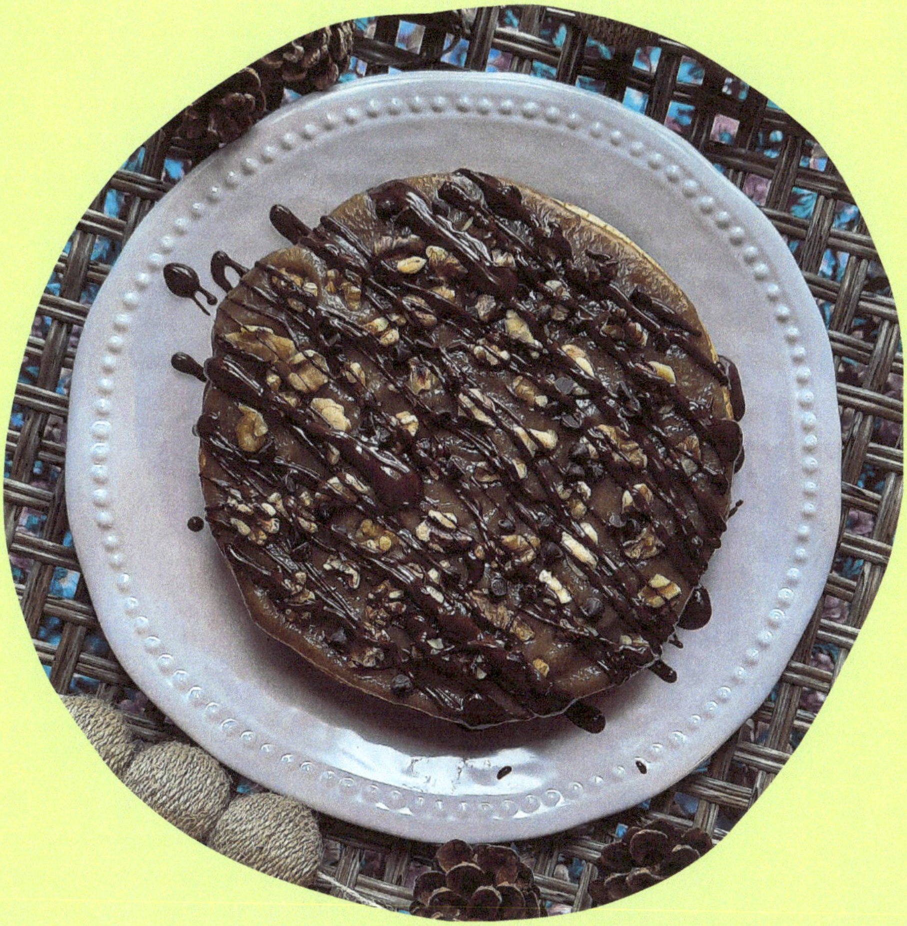

Chocolate Dream Cheesecake

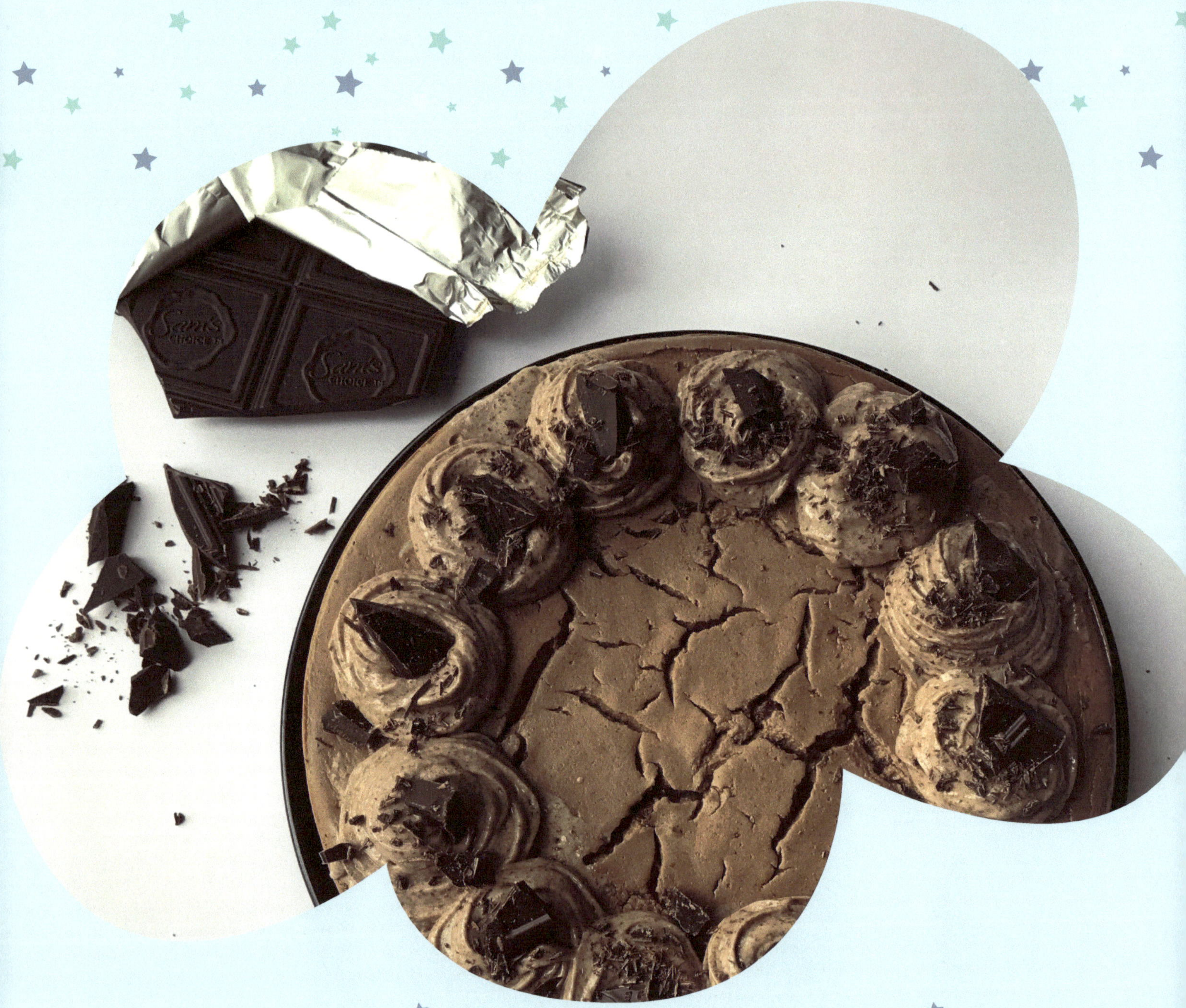

chocolate + cheesecake = a dream come true

Chocolate Dream Cheesecake

Crust Recipe:

- 2/3 c quick oats
- 1 tsp cocoa powder
- 1 tbsp honey
- 2 tbsp water

Crust Method:

- Stir all ingredients together
- Spray pan with oil
- Press crust into pan
- Wrap the bottom of the pan in a double layer of aluminum foil

Cheesecake Recipe:

- 1 c cottage cheese
- 8 oz fat free cream cheese
- 1/2 c vanilla greek yogurt
- 2 eggs
- 1/4 c honey
- 1 tbsp oats
- 1 tsp vanilla extract
- 1/2 c chocolate chips, melted (I used dark chocolate)
- chocolate chunks (measure with your heart)

Cheesecake Method:

- Add all ingredients except chocolate chunks to a food processor and blend until smooth
- Stir in chocolate chunks
- Pour cheesecake batter onto crust
- Cover cheesecake with aluminum foil
- Add water, lifting rack, and then cheesecake to pressure cooker
- Pressure cook on high for 35 minutes
- Wait for the pressure pin to release naturally
- Let cheesecake cool and refrigerate 8 hours or overnight before serving

Chocolate Dream Cheesecake

Chocolate Cream Cheese Frosting

Frosting Recipe:

- 8 oz fat free cream cheese
- 1/2 c to 1c confectioners sugar (can adjust to your desired sweetness level)
- 1/4 c chocolate chips melted (I used dark chocolate)

Frosting Method:

- Let cream cheese come to room temp
- Use a hand mixer to beat cream cheese
- While beating, add in sugar a little at a time
- While beating, add in melted chocolate
-Refrigerate

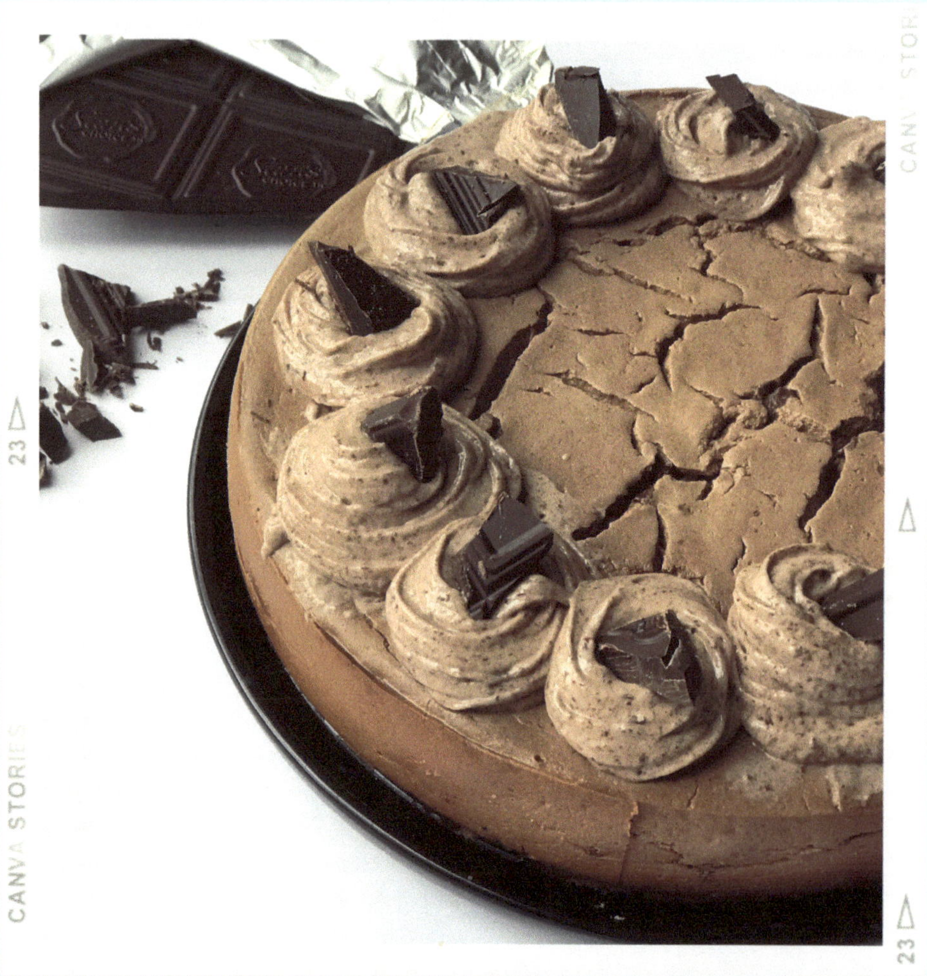

Assembly:

- Use a piping bag and star tip to pipe little swirls of frosting onto the edges of the cheesecake
- Top with more chocolate
- Devour :)

Lemon Poppy Seed Cheesecake

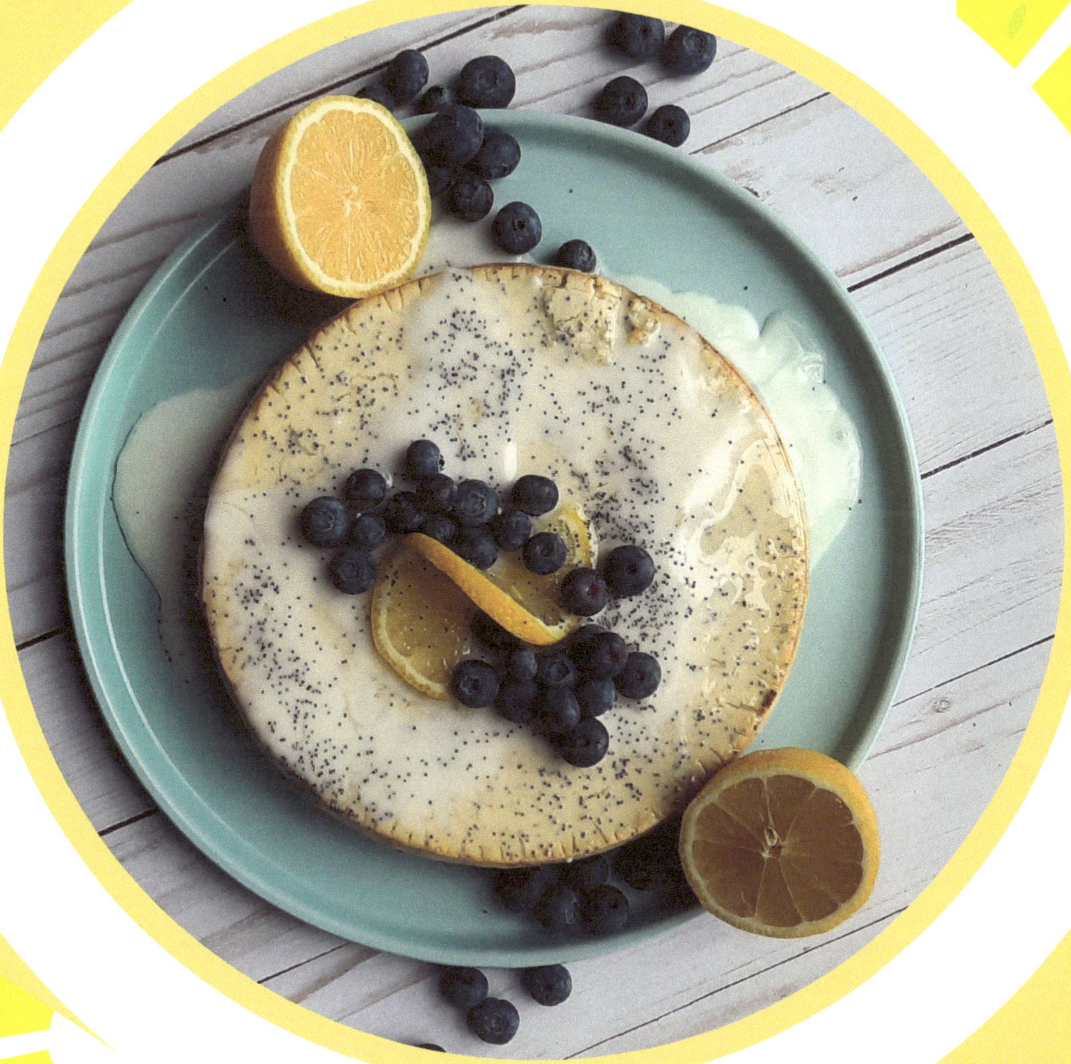

Light & Fruity!

Lemon Poppy Seed Cheesecake

Crust Recipe:

- 2/3 c quick oats
- 1 tbsp honey
- 2 tbsp water

Crust Method:

- Stir all ingredients together
- Spray pan with oil
- Press crust into pan
- Wrap the bottom of the pan in a double layer of aluminum foil

Cheesecake Recipe:

- 1 c cottage cheese
- 8 oz block fat free cream cheese
- 1/2 c vanilla greek yogurt
- 2 eggs
- 1/4 c honey
- 1 tbsp oats
- 1 tsp vanilla extract
- 1/2 tsp lemon zest (abt 1 lemon)
- 2 tsp lemon juice
- 1 tbsp poppy seeds

Cheesecake Method:

- Add all ingredients except poppy seeds to a food processor and blend until smooth
- Stir in poppy seeds
- Pour cheesecake batter onto crust
- Cover cheesecake with aluminum foil
- Add water, lifting rack, and then cheesecake to pressure cooker
- Pressure cook on high for 35 minutes
- Wait for the pressure pin to release naturally
- Let cheesecake cool and refrigerate 8 hours or overnight before serving

Lemon Poppy Seed Cheesecake

Glaze Recipe:

- 1 c powdered sugar
- 2 tsp fresh lemon juice
- 2 to 3 tsp water as needed, or more lemon juice for a stronger lemon flavor

Glaze Method:

- Stir sugar and lemon juice together
- Add water as needed to reach desired consistency
- Store at room temperature

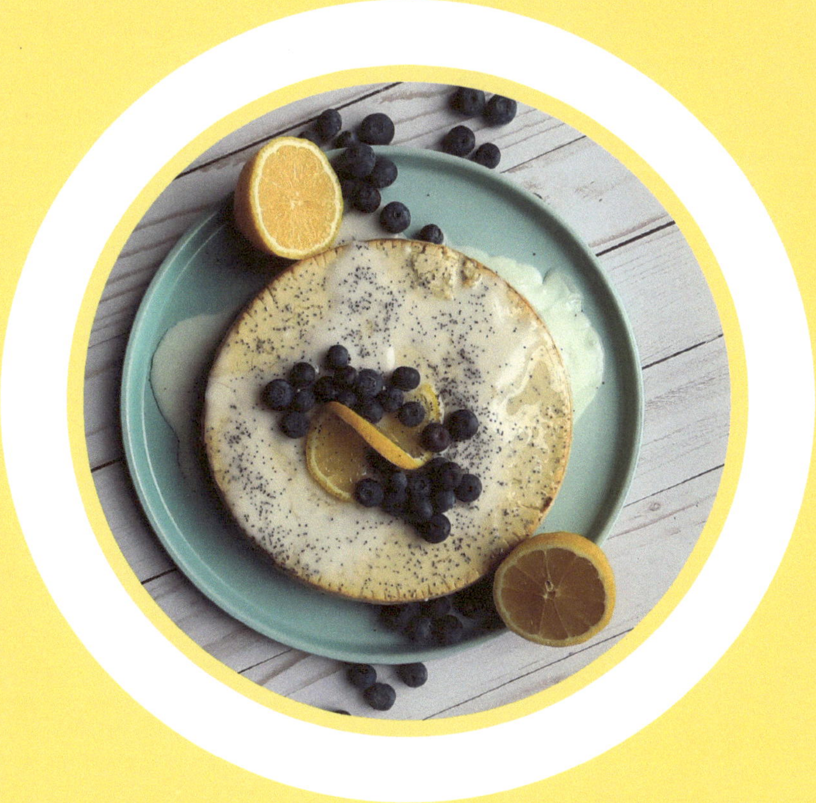

Assembly:

- Pour glaze over chilled cheesecake
- Add blueberries or other fruit
- Devour :)

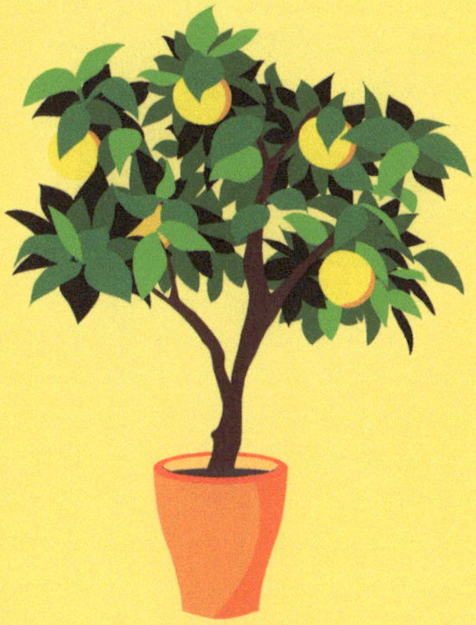

Chocolate Peppermint Cheesecake

Minty Bliss

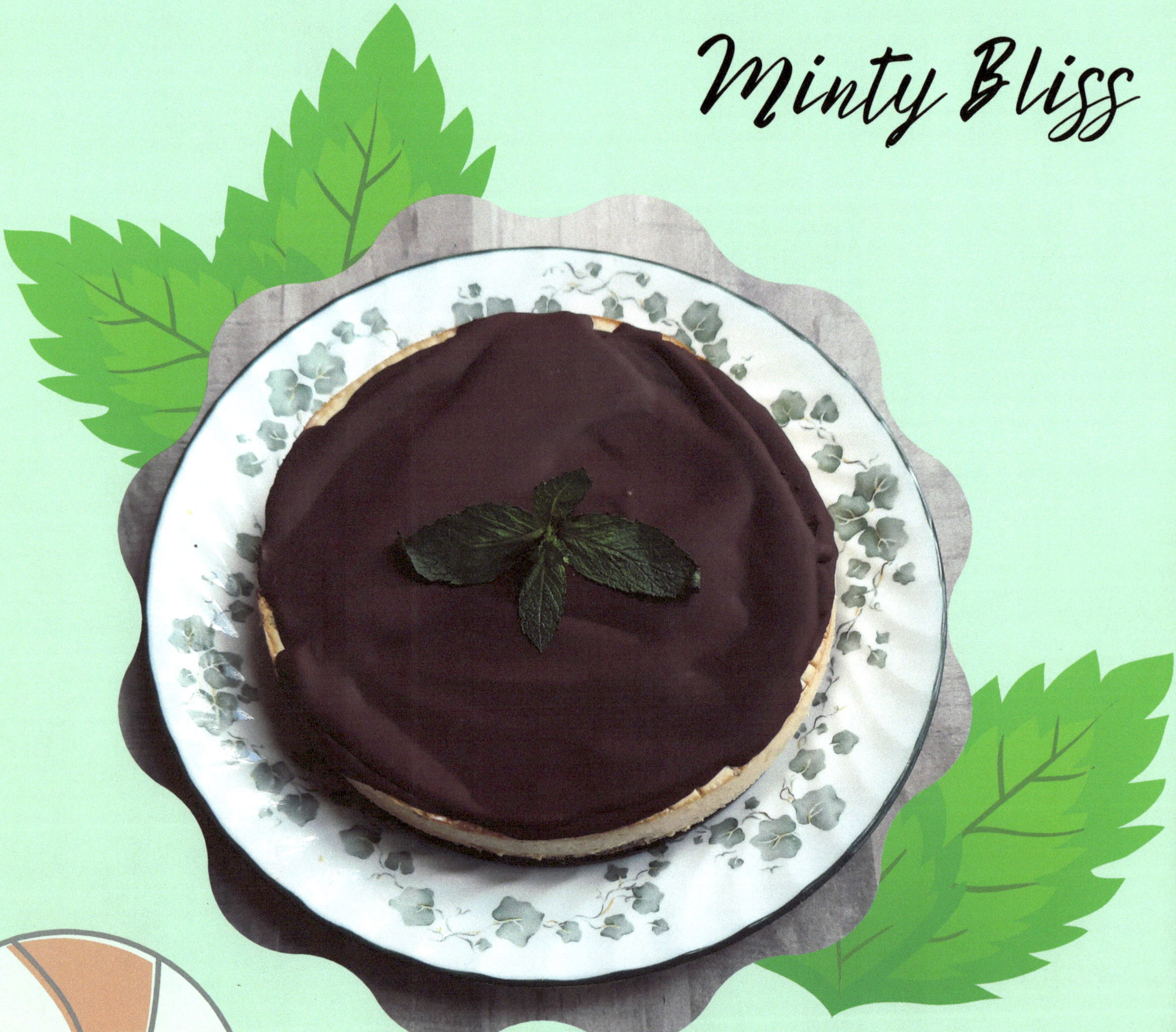

Chocolate Peppermint Cheesecake

Crust Recipe:

- 2/3 c quick oats
- 1 tsp cocoa powder
- 1 tbsp honey
- 2 tbsp water

Crust Method:

- Stir all ingredients together
- Spray pan with oil
- Press crust into pan
- Wrap the bottom of the pan in a double layer of aluminum foil

Cheesecake Recipe:

- 1 c cottage cheese
- 8 oz block fat free cream cheese
- 1/2 c vanilla greek yogurt
- 2 eggs
- 1/4 c honey
- 1 tbsp oats
- 1 tsp vanilla extract
- 1/4 tsp peppermint extract

Cheesecake Method:

- Add all ingredients to a food processor and blend until smooth
- Pour cheesecake batter onto crust
- Cover cheesecake with aluminum foil
- Add water, lifting rack, and then cheesecake to pressure cooker
- Pressure cook on high for 35 minutes
- Wait for the pressure pin to release naturally
- Let cheesecake cool and refrigerate 8 hours or overnight before serving

Chocolate Topping & Assembly

- Melt 1 c chocolate of choice
- Pour over top of cooled cheesecake
- Devour :)

Gingerbread Cheesecake

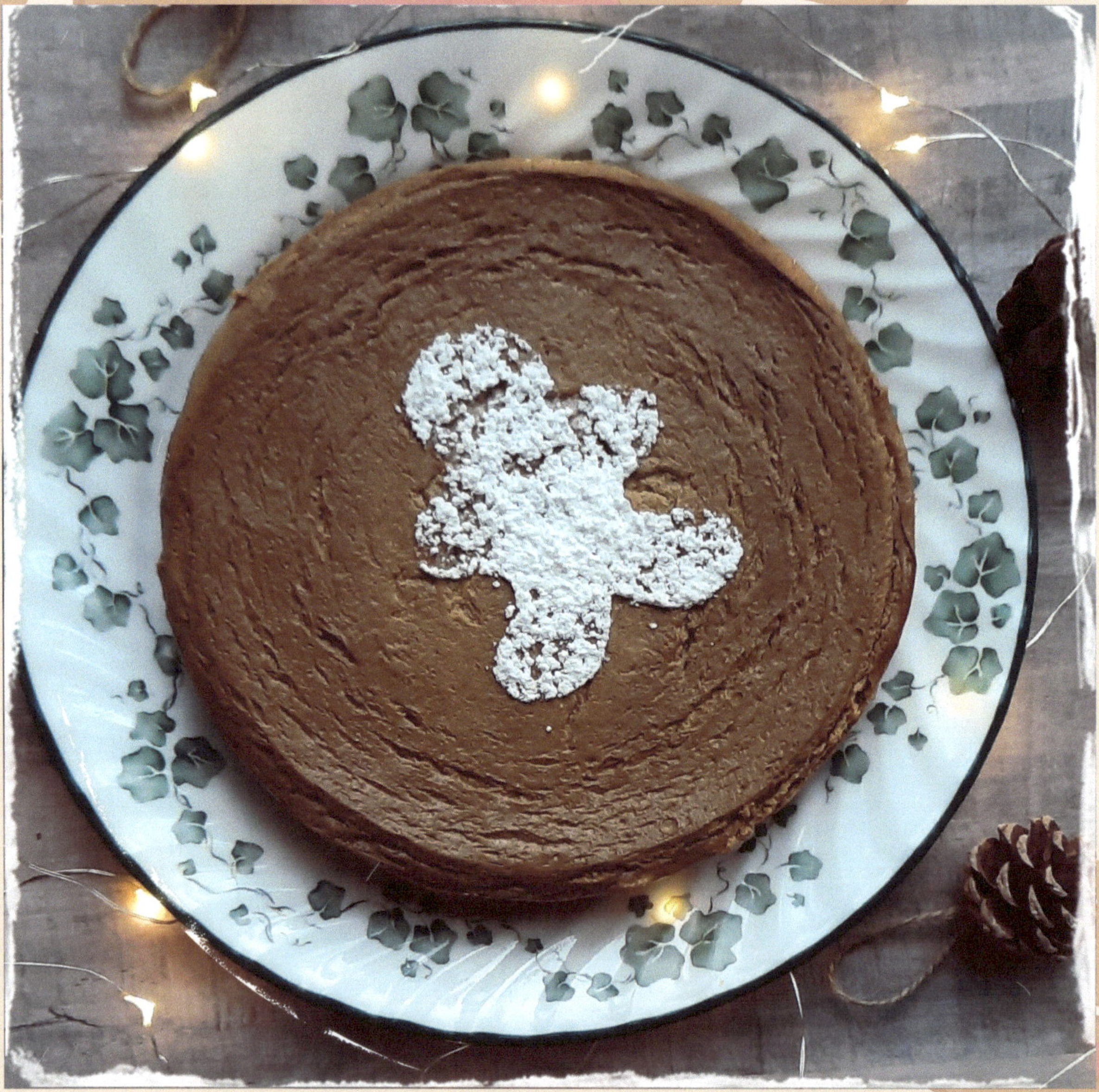

a classic holiday treat

Gingerbread Cheesecake

Crust Recipe:

- 2/3 c quick oats
- 1/4 tsp cinnamon
- 1 tbsp honey
- 2 tbsp water

Crust Method:

- Stir all ingredients together
- Spray pan with oil
- Press crust into pan
- Wrap the bottom of the pan in a double layer of aluminum foil

Cheesecake Recipe:

- 1 c cottage cheese
- 8 oz block fat free cream cheese
- 1/2 c vanilla greek yogurt
- 2 eggs
- 1/4 c molasses
- 1 tbsp oats
- 1 tsp vanilla extract
- 3/4 tsp ginger
- 3/4 tsp cinnamon
- 1/4 tsp nutmeg

Cheesecake Method:

- Add all ingredients to a food processor and blend until smooth
- Pour cheesecake batter onto crust
- Cover cheesecake with aluminum foil
- Add water, lifting rack, and then cheesecake to pressure cooker
- Pressure cook on high for 35 minutes
- Wait for the pressure pin to release naturally
- Let cheesecake cool and refrigerate 8 hours or overnight before serving
- Devour :)

Decorations!

- Cut a gingerbread shape out of a piece of paper
- Use the big piece as a template
- Sprinkle on powdered sugar
- Devour :)

Thank You!

I am so honored that you have purchased my first cookbook and tried the recipes!

It would mean so much to me if you reached out! My Instagram is @samantha.eatz
Please DM me any questions, comments, or concerns!

If you enjoyed these recipes please leave a book review!

Thank you again for showing me some love :)

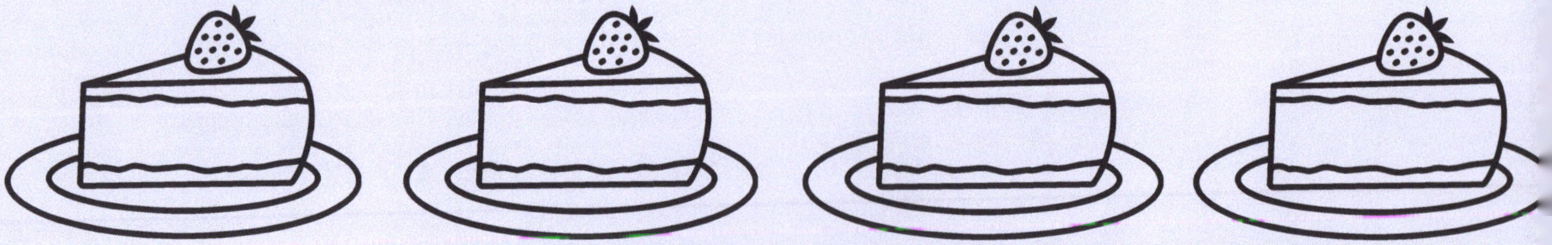